AF480142

With You, But Alone

How Loneliness Within Relationships Develops & How Connection is Restored

Dr. Jose Garcia-Cuellar
DSW, LCSW-S, CPT

© With You, But Alone

Published by Jose Garcia-Cuellar.

Copyright ©2026 Jose Garcia-Cuellar. All rights reserved.

All content in this book including, images, quotes, trademarks, processes, and logos are subject to copyright laws and trademark from the United States of America.

Any resemblance to any individual or group of characters in this book is a complete coincidence.

This book may not be reproduced in any form without the permission from the publisher or author.

ISBN: 979-8-9850818-9-3

JOSE GARCIA-CUELLAR, Author

WITH YOU, BUT ALONE

JOSE GARCIA-CUELLAR, DSW, LCSW-S, CPT

All rights reserved by Jose Garcia-Cuellar

The book is printed in the United States.

www.josegarciacuellar.com

Acknowledgments

This book would not exist without the relationships that shaped me the ones that held me, and the ones that didn't. To the clients who allowed me to witness their reaching, their loneliness, and their hope for connection, thank you for trusting me. Your experiences informed this work in ways that can never fully be named. To the people in my life who have shown me what reciprocal engagement feels like, and to those who unknowingly taught me what it does not thank you for shaping my understanding of connection. And to you, the reader: if you are here because something felt off, something felt lonely, or something needed words, this book is for you. Finally, to my daughter, may I continue to meet your bids for as long as I am alive. We all deserve to feel loved in the ways that matter to us.

Disclaimer

This book is intended for educational and reflective purposes only. It is not a substitute for psychotherapy, medical care, psychiatric treatment, or professional mental health advice. While the concepts, frameworks, and reflections shared in these pages are informed by clinical experience, research, and neuroscience-based perspectives, they are offered to support self-awareness and understanding, not diagnosis or treatment. Reading this book may bring up emotional responses, memories, or insights related to your relationships, attachment experiences, or sense of connection. This is a normal and human response when exploring topics related to intimacy, loneliness, and emotional safety. If at any point you find yourself feeling overwhelmed, distressed, or unsure how to process what is arising, it is encouraged that you seek support from a qualified mental health professional.

The frameworks described in this book, including Contact Loneliness, Reacher types, nervous system states, and the Reciprocity of Engagement Scale, are meant to offer language and perspective, not labels or judgments. They are not intended to define you, your partner, or your relationships in fixed or permanent ways. Human connection is dynamic, context-dependent, and influenced by many factors, including stress, health, history, and environment. Examples and reflections throughout this book may resemble real-life experiences, but they are presented for illustrative purposes only. Any resemblance to specific individuals or relationships is unintentional.

Finally, this book does not tell you what decisions to make about your relationships. Instead, it invites you to listen more closely to your own experience, your body, and your nervous system. Awareness is offered as a starting point, not a conclusion. You are encouraged to move at your own pace, with compassion for yourself and others, as you engage with this material.

A Note to the Reader

This book explores emotional connection, loneliness within relationships, and the ways our nervous systems adapt when connection is inconsistent. Some sections may bring up feelings, memories, or realizations about your own relationships, past or present. You are encouraged to read at your own pace. You may want to pause, reflect, journal, or return to sections later. All of that is welcome.

If at any point the material feels overwhelming, activating, or emotionally heavy, consider taking a break and doing something regulating for your body, such as stepping outside, slowing your breath, or grounding yourself in the present moment. Reaching out for professional support is also a valid and supported choice. This book is not meant to push you toward confrontation, decisions, or conclusions before you are ready. It is meant to help you notice patterns with clarity and compassion, and to offer language for experiences that are often felt but rarely identified. One more thing, this book is meant to be helpful for both individuals in that relationship. It is intended to promote awareness and understanding of how responding to each other can promote either bonding or loneliness without blaming or villanizing.

How to Use This Book

This book is designed to be both informative and experiential. While it can be read straight through, it is also meant to be returned to over time. As you read, consider the following:

- *Read slowly, especially if you notice strong emotional reactions.*

- *Pay attention not only to what you think, but to what you feel in your body.*

- *Notice moments of recognition without rushing to label or judge yourself.*

- *Allow insights to unfold without forcing action or change.*

The reflection and journaling sections are optional but encouraged. They are not assignments. You may choose to write, think quietly, or simply notice what arises. At the end of the book, The Reciprocity of Engagement Scale is included as a tool for awareness. It is meant to help clarify patterns over time, not to prove something or assign fault. You do not need to act on your results immediately, or at all. Sometimes understanding is the intervention. Most importantly, this book is not asking you to become less emotional, less relational, or less needing of connection. It is helping you understand *why* connection has felt the way it has, and what conditions allow it to feel safer, more mutual, and more sustaining.

Contents

Chapter 1

Contact Loneliness

Have you ever felt lonely within a relationship? This kind of loneliness can be hard to identify. There is a difference between being alone and feeling lonely. Alone is a physical state in which there is no one around you, and the other is an emotional state of feeling isolated or disconnected. Throughout this book, I refer to this experience as *Contact Loneliness*. This describes the experience of feeling emotionally alone despite ongoing interaction, communication, or proximity. It develops not from absence or neglect, but from repeated moments of being responded to without being emotionally met. Over time, these near-misses shape how safe it feels to reach, connect, and remain emotionally engaged. Contact Loneliness develops from being almost met.

It shows up in interactions that continue, but don't quite leave you feeling seen, settled, or connected. Perhaps you might walk away feeling a sense of sadness or disappointment and unsure of why. Perhaps it is because the other person just couldn't quite match your "vibe or energy," or because they were physically present but emotionally absent, as if going through the motions but not fully engaging. These interactions feel close enough to keep you going, but not close enough to feel connected.

Many people carry this kind of loneliness because, on the surface, they may be surrounded by caring individuals. There are relationships, conversations, routines, and people who respond when they reach out. No one is obviously absent, and yet something still feels missing, and it might feel difficult to explain. This can be especially confusing because nothing seems "wrong," so who or what is to blame? Overall, there may be care, goodwill, and even consistency. People show up and they respond with good intentions. Still, after certain interactions, you might notice a familiar feeling, a sense of disappointment, distance instead of closeness, or empty instead of full. Over time, this can leave you feeling disconnected, discouraged, disappointed, and worn down.

If this is a familiar feeling, as a reminder to you, this does not mean you are asking for too much, and you are not imagining something that isn't there. Many people experience Contact Loneliness because their moments of connection within certain relationships don't reliably offer the kind of emotional meeting that helps the body relax and the heart feel held or connected. Most of us were never taught to recognize this difference. Personally, it took me years to finally identify and name how Contact Loneliness shaped my day-to-day interactions. We may have learned how to respond to one another, to reply, to listen, to engage, but we're rarely taught how emotional connection works. More importantly, we aren't taught how timing matters, how emotional energy matters, or how much the body pays attention to whether an interaction feels regulating or draining. So, when connection falls short, we often turn inward, assuming the problem must be us or feeling as if we are unworthy of affection or love.

This book is an invitation to challenge that assumption. Throughout these pages, we'll look closely at the difference between being responded to and being emotionally met. We'll explore the small, often invisible moments that shape whether connection feels alive or hollow. And we'll name the ways people adapt over time, sometimes by reaching less, sometimes by working harder, sometimes by staying quiet when connection repeatedly misses. It offers language for experiences many people have had across their lives, not just in romantic relationships, but in friendships, families, work relationships, and everyday interactions. It explores how loneliness can develop even when people care, and how it can persist without neglect, conflict, or obvious rejection. This book is about understanding how interactions sometimes fail to meet the full bid of connection, why that hurts, and where awareness can begin to make space for something different. Not forced closeness or perfect communication, just moments that feel more settling, mutual, and attuned.

If you've spent years wondering why relationships feel tiring, distant, or lonely despite your best efforts, I hope this book provides you with a sense of relief, allowing you to finally feel seen and understood as to why Contact Loneliness has lingered in your life just as it has in mine. If you've been reaching for connection your whole life, let this book guide you to identifying what you're missing in those moments of connection and how to assess which relationships are reciprocating engagement and which ones are not. Additionally, it will help promote the cultivation of reciprocated relationships in hopes of reaching for healing. As a gentle reminder, this book applies to any relationship, (parents, siblings, coworkers, friends etc.) since bids are made in everyday life. However, for this book, we will be using romantic relationships as examples. Before we can truly understand the relational impacts of missed bids, let's understand what a bid is and then how the different nervous system states influence our day-to-day interactions.

Chapter 2

Attempts at Connection (Bids)

Have you ever wondered why it may be easier to feel seen by some people and not others? Or why certain relationships feel more connecting, even when the amount of communication looks similar? Most people don't think of themselves as reaching for connection. They're just talking, sharing, joking, venting, asking, or sitting next to someone they care about. And yet, beneath these ordinary moments are small, meaningful reaches. Brief moments that say, "Can you meet me here?" These reaches are often called bids.

A bid is any attempt, whether conscious or unconscious, to initiate emotional contact with another person. These attempts may take the form of a comment, a question, a look, a gesture, shared silence, or a shift in tone. Some bids are easy and playful. Others are tender, hesitant, or wrapped in everyday conversation, and can be direct or indirect. Gottman's research found that the success of relationships is not determined by the absence of conflict, but by how often partners turn toward bids for connection rather than turning away or against them (Gottman et al., 1998). However, turning toward a bid alone may not always feel reciprocated. Meaning, the more frequent bids are reciprocated and met, the closeness the relationship will feel. The opposite is also true, the more time spend turning away and not meeting or matching bids it can promote feelings of isolation, relational neglect, and other relational complications.

Through my clinical and personal experience, I noticed that even when someone turns toward a bid, it can still feel empty. Therefore, I like to introduce the *Bid-Response-Reciprocity Model (BRR)* which describes how emotional connection is built, maintained, or eroded through everyday interactions. A *bid* is an attempt to reach for connection. A *response* is how that bid is acknowledged or engaged. *Reciprocity* refers to whether the response arrives with enough presence, timing, and emotional alignment to settle the nervous system and sustain connection.

Connection does not depend on bids alone, nor on responses alone, but on the quality of reciprocity over time. When bids are responded to without being emotionally met, the body registers near-misses. Repeated near-misses shape nervous system adaptations, influence reaching patterns, and can gradually lead to Contact Loneliness within ongoing relationships. Essentially, the more these bids are fully met and reciprocated, the more positively it can impact the relationship. For example, some relationships may not argue but may also not connect to each other, thus creating distance of time or width within the relationship without truly cultivating depth. These relationships may feel surface level, whereas, others may feel as if you've known each other for so long because the bids are immediately met at their fullest, whereas in others, bids may be sporadic or infrequent, only allowing time to be the true connection to that relationship. Maybe you have a friend for ten years but aren't really that well connected, versus someone else you've known for one year and have a deeper relationship with. Does your relationship have distance or depth?

Turning toward a bid communicates availability, interest, and emotional presence, while repeated missed or dismissed bids predict emotional distance and relational dissatisfaction over time. This is how relationships begin to disconnect and erode connection. The true intention of a bid is not how dramatic or clear it is, but how it carries emotional energy while inviting a response. Every bid ask, in some way, "Is connection available right now?"

Outside of research or therapy spaces, that word can sound abstract or technical, but in everyday life, a bid is simple. It's any moment where you lean toward someone emotionally or physically, even shared silence, such as asking to sit next to each other quietly. Bids are attempts to test whether connection is available, and these interactions happen constantly throughout the day. You might not notice yourself making bids because they often feel automatic. You say, "You won't believe what happened today," or "Can I tell you something?" You send a meme, share a memory, reach for someone's hand, or sit a little closer on the couch. Or asking them to read this book with you. What makes these moments bids isn't the words themselves; it's the subconscious hope underneath them.

Every bid carries emotional energy. Some are light and easy, asking for shared attention or playfulness. Others are more vulnerable, asking for comfort, reassurance, or understanding. Others may be more direct or intense, and bids can appear across different levels of intimacy, including sexual interactions. But what happens when you find yourself constantly making bids to feel connected? It is important to note that making frequent bids is not a sign of neediness.

From early on, most of us learn through experience what happens when we reach. Over time, we notice who responds, how they respond, and whether those moments feel comforting or uncomfortable. This is one way we evaluate relationships. Some feel more exhausting than others, while one relationship might feel replenishing or giving, and other feels depleting and draining. Over time, these experiences shape how often we bid, how clearly, we bid, and how much we expect in return.

You may begin to recognize this in yourself. Perhaps you tend to reach openly and directly. Or maybe you soften your bids, couching them in humor or practicality. Some people explain more, hoping clarity will help the other person meet them. Others ask less, waiting to see if someone notices on their own. None of these patterns are wrong. They are adaptations developed to protect against Contact Loneliness.

What often goes unnoticed is that bids don't just ask for a response. They ask for emotional meeting. They ask for presence, timing, and emotional alignment. When a bid is met in a way that feels attuned, the nervous system and body settle. When it isn't, even if a response occurs, the body remembers and may register a negative response.

This is why people can find themselves reaching again and again, trying to adjust how they ask. And it's why others slowly stop reaching altogether, not because they don't care, but because the effort of reaching begins to outweigh the relief of connection. If you pause for a moment, you might start to notice these patterns in your own life.

Reflections

Before moving on, you may want to take a moment to notice how you tend to reach and receive:

- *When you want to feel closer to someone, what do you usually do?*

- *Do you reach openly and directly, or more quietly and indirectly?*

- *Are your bids playful, practical, emotional, or subtle?*

- *Have your bids changed over time in response to how others meet you?*

You might also reflect on how you **experience** responses:

- *Can you think of times when someone responded, but you still felt unseen?*

- *Are there people who say very little, yet leave you feeling calmer or more connected?*

- *After certain interactions, do you feel more settled or more drained?*

Finally, you might notice how you respond when others reach for you:

- *When someone bids for your attention or emotional presence, how available do you tend to be?*

- *Are there moments when you want to meet someone more fully, but feel limited by stress, fatigue, or distraction?*

- *How does it feel in your body when you're able to truly meet someone, and when you're not?*

There's nothing you need to do with these reflections right now other than notice and create space for awareness. As we move forward, we'll look more closely at what happens after a bid is made, how responses differ, why some moments land while others miss, and how patterns of closeness or loneliness quietly take shape without anyone intending them to. To understand why turning toward a bid doesn't always prevent loneliness, it helps to look at connection through a broader lens. This is where the Bid–Response–Reciprocity Model becomes useful. Now that you have language for what a bid really is, and why being responded to doesn't always mean being met, let's dive deeper into why saying yes or turning toward a bid may still fall short of connection.

Why Turning Toward Isn't Always Enough

Many people have been told that connection depends on whether someone responds. That if a partner, friend, or loved one turns toward you and answers your message, listens to your words, or stays engaged, then connection should naturally follow. This can be particularly difficult because they may respond with, "But I was there with you," or "I listened to what you had to say." But as you've likely noticed, that isn't always what happens. What matters isn't only whether someone responds to a bid, but the extent to which it is met and how that response is experienced. A response can acknowledge a reach without fully meeting it. Someone can turn toward you behaviorally while missing you emotionally.

The Body's Reaction to Not Being Met

When you reach for connection, something unfolds beneath the surface. First, there is the reach itself, the bid. This is the moment you lean toward someone emotionally, offering a feeling, a thought, or a need for shared presence. Then comes the response. The other person may either *turn toward* you, leaning into the bid with acceptance, *turn away* by rejecting, denying, or disengaging, or *turn against* the reach with a hostile or aggressive response. In many relationships, turning toward happens often enough that things continue on the surface. But here is the piece that has been unnamed. After the response, the nervous system subconsciously evaluates whether the interaction matched what was offered. Did the energy align within the appropriate time frame? Did the response arrive with the same emotional intensity? Was there enough presence to feel accompanied?

This is the moment where connection either settles or slips into relational misalignment. When a response matches the reach well enough, the body registers relief, a sense of feeling seen, felt, or understood. This can look like feeling relaxed, calm, or even excited. When it doesn't, even if someone turned toward you, the reach could still feel unmet. Over time, repeated experiences like this shape how safe it feels to keep reaching at all. This is exactly how Contact Loneliness develops, through repeated bids that are met, but emotionally absent. Just because someone agreed to accept the bid doesn't mean they reciprocated the engagement.

This is why turning toward on its own isn't always enough to prevent loneliness. Responsiveness keeps interaction going. Ultimately, reciprocal engagement is what makes connection land. When reciprocal engagement is inconsistent, the body adapts, often without words, without conflict, and without blame. These inconsistent responses or misaligned reaches become a pattern, resulting in emotional distance within the relationship.

Contact Loneliness rarely begins with a single moment. It forms gradually through patterns that are easy to miss while they are happening. Most people don't wake up one day and decide to stop reaching. They don't consciously choose distance. Instead, Contact Loneliness grows through repeated experiences of almost being met, almost being understood, and almost feeling connected. Over time, the body, or nervous system, learns from these moments, even when the mind tries to explain them away. When bids are met inconsistently, when energy doesn't quite match, or when timing or presence feels limited, the nervous system adapts. Not dramatically, but subtly. It begins to conserve and becomes more careful to prevent emotional injury. It reaches a little less freely. This is how missing becomes a pattern.

Why Energy Mismatches Hurt

Energy matching is about emotional proximity, coming close enough to the emotional tone of the bid that the other person feels accompanied rather than alone. Have you ever wondered how often you or your partner pause and sense what the other person is bringing into the interaction?

When energy isn't matched, people adapt without realizing it. Connection is not just emotional, but deeply biological. Every bid for connection is processed by the nervous system as information, not just what happened, but whether the experience felt settling, relieving, effortful, or costly. Over time, these experiences shape the social brain, the body's stress responses, and the felt sense of safety in relationship. The social brain is a network of regions in the brain that processes social cues, intention, and tracks closeness and belonging, regulating through relationship. It evaluates this information and translates it into nervous system responses that help us bond, feel safe, repair disconnection, or brace when connection feels uncertain. These processes shape bonding, motivation, trust, and the capacity to stay emotionally engaged with others.

Understanding this can offer a different narrative for how to interpret missed interactions. Contact Loneliness is impacted by another person's response. These are biological responses to relational conditions. Over time, the body may begin to tense or guard, learning implicitly and often unconsciously that reaching carries risk. It is also important to recognize that energy mismatches aren't always intentional. There are many factors that impact how someone responds or how available they are to a bid. Stress, exhaustion, distraction, and overwhelm can limit a person's capacity to meet another emotionally in the moment. Someone may care deeply and still struggle to match energy consistently. Understanding this can reduce blame without dismissing impact.

From a relational and nervous system perspective, Contact Loneliness reflects repeated disruptions in reciprocal engagement where energy, timing, or presence do not align closely enough for the body to register safety and connection. Although relationships may remain active and intact on the surface, the nervous system adapts to these subtle misses by conserving, mobilizing, or staying vigilant, ultimately sustaining loneliness within contact and resulting in feeling lonely within the relationship.

Adapting for Protection

When connection repeatedly fails to land, the nervous system looks for ways to protect itself. For some people, this looks like reaching less. For others, it looks like reaching harder by explaining more, pushing for clarity, or asking directly for reassurance. Over time, however, these adaptations can change the dynamics of a relationship. Emotional conversations become rarer. Bids become smaller or more practical. Vulnerability is postponed. What once felt alive begins to feel functional. Contact Loneliness arrives slowly, in the space between interactions that continue but no longer nourish.

One of the hardest parts of this type of loneliness is that it often exists alongside care, consistency, and goodwill. People may still show up reliably. They may still communicate. They may even believe the relationship is healthy, while the other person might believe the complete opposite. This isn't miscommunication. It is a misalignment in connection. This makes the loneliness harder to trust and understand. "I shouldn't feel lonely if my partner is with me." Many people tell themselves they shouldn't feel this way. Nothing is wrong. They're trying. I shouldn't complain. And so, the feeling goes unnamed, carried privately, sometimes for years or even a lifetime. But Contact Loneliness doesn't require neglect to take root. It only requires repeated experiences where emotional reaching doesn't reliably land with the full components. Not fully meeting a bid creates in emotional distance.

When Reaching Feels Risky

As these patterns settle in, something important shifts. Reaching begins to feel less natural and more effortful. The body remembers previous misses and anticipates them. The nervous system becomes cautious, even in the presence of care. You may find yourself at the brink of making a bid but immediately withholding or choosing not to make it because something in your body doesn't feel right.

This is often when people begin to say things like:

- *"I just don't feel close anymore."*

- *"We talk, but it feels surface level."*

- *"I don't know why I feel lonely. I'm not alone."*

- *"I should be grateful for their presence."*

These are signals of unmet emotional rhythms over time.

Reflections

You might take a moment to reflect on how patterns of missing have shaped your own relationships:

- *Have you noticed yourself reaching less over time in certain relationships?*

- *Are there parts of yourself you no longer bring forward because it feels tiring or risky?*

- *Do you feel more emotionally alone now than you did earlier in the relationship, even though things still function?*

- *How does your body respond when you consider reaching again?*

Again, this is a reminder to simply sit and notice your responses. In the next chapter, we'll look more closely at the specific ways people adapt when connection becomes uncertain or inconsistent. We'll explore the different ways people learn to reach, how some become quieter, some try harder, and some stay vigilant, so you can better understand how your own reaching has been shaped and why it has always made sense. Over time, when bids land inconsistently, miss emotionally, or feel unsafe to offer, people don't stop wanting connection. They adapt how they reach for it. These adaptations are rarely conscious, and they're not personality flaws. They are the nervous system's way of protecting closeness while trying to reduce pain.

Four Reacher Types

How We Adapt When Connection Is Inconsistent

When emotional meeting becomes inconsistent, people don't stop wanting connection. Over time, they adapt how they reach for it. It is important to remember that these Reacher types are not personality traits or character flaws. They are purely adaptive and fluid. As we review the four different Reacher types, I encourage you to think about your relationships. You might find that you reach differently depending on the person or may fluctuate between reaching types within the same relationship over time. This is important because these patterns offer information about how others respond to your bids, and whether those responses feel reciprocated, safe, or unsafe.

Reacher types are behaviors developed as protective strategies in which the nervous system has learned to preserve closeness while reducing emotional cost. The result is four common patterns that tend to emerge. People may move between them across different relationships or life stages, and these patterns can change depending on the person.

These patterns are:

- *Collapsed Reaching (protects self by conserving and reaching less)*

- *Mobilized Reaching (protects self by escalating and reaching more)*

- *Vigilant Reaching (protects by monitoring)*

- *Secure Reaching (reciprocated trust and reaching safely)*

Each reflects a different response to the same underlying question: *Is it safe, and is it worth it to keep reaching?*

As a reminder, being responded to means a bid was turned toward, accepted, and acknowledged. Being emotionally met means the bid was received with enough presence, timing, and emotional alignment or attunement to settle the nervous system. When bids are emotionally met consistently, reaching feels natural and safe. When they are met inconsistently or not at all, the nervous system adapts.

Collapsed Reacher

The person who adapts by reaching less Over time, when moments of being emotionally met are rare or inconsistent, some people become Collapsed Reachers. They stop reaching as much, lower their expectations, and begin to feel as though they themselves are "too much" or are asking for too much. Energy lowers. Reaching becomes quieter. Emotional needs are pushed inward. What often follows is sadness, loneliness, and the slow development of negative self-beliefs within the relationship. Importantly, some people don't reach less because they are naturally quiet. They reach less because it stopped feeling safe to reach at all. Motivation to initiate connection decreases. "I don't feel like reaching anymore," even though they still long for closeness.

When Reaching Stops Feeling Safe

Up to this point, we've been talking about how people adapt their reaching when connection is inconsistent or emotionally thin. But there is another important reason people may grow quieter over time, one that has less to do with disappointment and more to do with safety. Sometimes people stop reaching because it no longer feels safe to make a bid. In relationships that feel unpredictable, controlling, critical, or emotionally volatile, bids for connection can carry risk. A bid may be turned away, ignored, or dismissed, or more harmfully, turned against the person and later used with blame, deflection, or ridicule.

Eventually, the nervous system learns that reaching doesn't just fail to connect but can create harm. Due to these hostile interactions, the Reacher may suppress bids as a means of survival or protection. People may begin to internalize their needs, telling themselves they shouldn't want more or shouldn't need connection at all. They may become quieter, more self-contained, or emotionally guarded. In these dynamics, becoming a Collapsed Reacher is a survival strategy.

This kind of adaptation is especially common in relationships marked by emotional manipulation, chronic invalidation, coercive control, or repeated boundary violations. However, it can also occur in subtler ways, such as when expressing needs reliably leads to conflict, dismissal, or emotional fallout. Withholding bids in unsafe relationships is an adaptation to the relational environment and should not be mistaken for poor communication.

Understanding this distinction matters, because the path forward is different. When reaching has been shaped by unsafety, the work is not about reaching more. It is about restoring internal and relational safety before connection can feel possible again. This can take time and a great deal of self-awareness from both individuals. In conclusion, not all Collapsed Reachers develop from disappointment. Sometimes, they develop from dangerous or harmful relationships.

Core experience: This pattern protects by minimizing emotional cost:

- *Learns that reaching isn't reliable or safe.*

- *Turns the volume down on needs and expression.*

- *Begins to feel burdensome or "too much".*

- *Loses spontaneity, energy, and emotional ease.*

- *Internalizes sadness, loneliness, and self-doubt.*

Supporting Research: Collapsed Reaching

Research across attachment theory, emotion regulation, and neurobiology suggests that some individuals adapt to relational inconsistency by reducing their bids for connection. This does not reflect a lack of desire for closeness, but rather a learned strategy to minimize emotional cost. Attachment researchers describe deactivating strategies as ways individuals protect themselves when closeness feels unreliable, intrusive, or overwhelming. In these cases, people downregulate emotional expression, suppress attachment needs, and rely more heavily on self-sufficiency (Fraley & Shaver, 2000; Mikulincer & Shaver, 2016). Collapsed reaching can reflect this same protective process. In everyday life, it may look like reaching less, needing less, at least on the surface, or going quiet, not because connection doesn't matter, but because wanting it has begun to feel dysregulating.

Emotion regulation research supports this pattern, showing that repeated experiences of unmet emotional responses increase expressive suppression. While suppression may reduce immediate distress, it often comes at the cost of emotional vitality and felt connection (Gross,

2015). From a nervous system perspective, collapsed reaching reflects a shift toward conservation. When reaching repeatedly fails to bring relief or regulation, the body learns to lower emotional volume to reduce disappointment. Importantly, this pattern may emerge as a long-standing attachment strategy or as a situational response within specific relationships where emotional unsafety, inconsistency, or repeated mismatch has occurred.

Mobilized Reacher

On other occasions, some may respond to inconsistent connection by doing the opposite. They become mobilized. They begin to explain more and become more direct with their bids. Mobilized Reachers tend to work harder to be understood and to increase a sense of connection. They increase effort in hopes that clarity, persistence, or emotional labor will help the connection land. However, over time, this constant reaching can become exhausting. It also cultivates a sense of one-sided relationships. The result is emotional burnout. If you find yourself constantly thinking of ways to connect with your partner and intentionally reaching more, while becoming frustrated that your partner is not reaching as often as you, then this is you adapting.

This can happen if the other person is already a Collapsed Reacher and you find yourself trying to connect, so you become more effortful in your bids or reach more often to get a response from your partner. The challenge here is that this later becomes a form of enabling. The connection feels heavier to carry because only one person sees themselves as solely responsible for maintaining it. Therefore, instead of encouraging the receiving partner to reach more, we reinforce their passive approach. The real issue here is fear from the Mobilized Reacher. Ask yourself this: "If I stop reaching, do I fear we won't be connected?" What often follows is frustration, anger, resentment, and painful beliefs about being unwanted or unworthy of love. For some, the lack of reciprocity may translate into the belief that the other person doesn't care enough, and therefore doesn't desire them, love them, or feel interested in them.

Core experience: This pattern protects by increasing effort:

- *Tries harder to be understood.*

- *Explains more and asks more directly.*

- *Carries most of the emotional labor.*

- *Becomes burned out, exhausted, resentful, and frustrated.*

- *Begins to feel unwanted, rejected, misunderstood, and unworthy.*

Supporting Research: Mobilized Reaching

Attachment research describes a hyperactivating strategy, where individuals respond to perceived unavailability by intensifying proximity-seeking behaviors (Cassidy & Berlin, 1994; Mikulincer & Shaver, 2016). Emotion regulation research shows that when emotional needs are inconsistently met, individuals may increase expression and explanation in an effort to secure understanding (Gross, 2015). While this can temporarily increase connection, it often places a disproportionate emotional burden on the Reacher.

Interpersonal research suggests that carrying unequal emotional labor over time leads to fatigue and resentment (Butler, 2011). From a nervous system perspective, mobilized reaching reflects sustained activation. The body stays oriented toward repair and reassurance, which maintains engagement but can make true settling difficult. It also depletes internal resources, lowering mental and emotional capacity. It is important to remember that Mobilized Reaching is not neediness, but persistence for connection.

Vigilant Reacher

Vigilant Reachers are, in my opinion, one of the most detrimental patterns to the nervous system. When bids are fully met but not reliably, the nervous system can become stuck in a painful in-between state. The Vigilant Reacher does not fully stop reaching, because connection does happen and is reciprocated at times. Bids may be fully met by the receiver with all the necessary components, but the Reacher cannot relax into it because they do not know when it will happen again. This is the hardest part. Knowing that your partner has the capacity to fully meet your bid, and that it feels amazing when they do, but that it is so sporadic or inconsistent keeps the Reacher wondering, "Will my bid be met this time?"

You may make a bid one time, and it is fully met, and the next time, even the same type of bid may be almost met. This makes it difficult to know when and what bids will be met. This creates uncertainty within the relationship and results in a hypervigilant state of alert. The result is a pattern of staying emotionally on call, hopeful, alert, yet lonely during in-between periods of time, vigilantly waiting for the next fully reciprocated experience. This can also be understood as breadcrumbing, when the receiver gives just enough to keep you holding on to hope, yet not enough to feel fulfilled or satisfied.

This pattern is exhausting. Constantly making bids and coming up short, and then having a bid fully met, can create confusion. In the receiver's mind, it may be interpreted as, "Well, I did what you asked the other day," or "I was there, so you should feel appreciative." However, the lack of consistency begins to feel conflicting and unsettling. This vigilant response also comes with physical reactions. Your body might tense, and you may experience anxiety related to not knowing whether your bid is safe to make. In addition, you might find yourself spiraling or cycling through past bids, trying to figure out why some bids are fully met and why others are only almost met. The Reacher may fluctuate in their reaching, sometimes reaching more and other times reaching less, while also waiting for the other person to make efforts to connect. Over time, this overwhelms the nervous system.

Core experience: This pattern protects by staying close enough to experience connection, while bracing for loss:

- *Gets just enough connection to keep hope alive.*

- *Feels stuck in "maybe," waiting, and uncertainty.*

- *Becomes hypervigilant to tone, timing, and closeness.*

- *Replays interactions and searches for meaning.*

- *Feels lonely while still emotionally invested.*

- *Over time, may protect through emotional numbing.*

Supporting Research: Vigilant Reaching

Attachment research shows that inconsistent responsiveness uniquely amplifies insecurity. When availability is unpredictable, the nervous system becomes more alert rather than disengaged (Cassidy & Berlin, 1994). More recent research shows that variability in responsiveness predicts attachment anxiety more strongly than average responsiveness alone (Günaydin et al., 2021). Whitchurch et al. (2011) note how uncertainty increases cognitive preoccupation and emotional vigilance, which helps explain why Vigilant Reachers remain invested while feeling unsettled. Over time, sustained vigilance can become exhausting. Research suggests prolonged uncertainty may eventually lead to emotional numbing or deactivation as a protective response

(Simpson, 2017). From a nervous system perspective, Vigilant Reaching reflects orientation without safety. The body stays close and may literally tense to brace for disappointment.

Secure Reacher

Finally, we have the Secure Reacher. There is hope, y'all. When bids for connection are met with the full components of enough consistency, presence, and emotional alignment, a different pattern of reaching can emerge. This person reaches without bracing, withdrawing, or over-efforting. The trust to reach is implicit, and connection is available because reaching will not require self-abandonment or self-protection. There is something that relaxes within us; our bodies feel at ease and lighter knowing a bid was fully met and reciprocated.

The Secure Reacher does not monitor connection constantly, nor do they minimize their needs to avoid disappointment. They also don't escalate effort to secure closeness. Instead, they reach openly and flexibly, adjusting naturally to the moment and the relationship. This pattern develops not because connection has been perfect, but because it has been reliably good enough and reciprocated. The key here is reciprocity of engagement. This allows the relationship to feel balanced by promoting mutual interest and an even transfer of emotional energy.

This relationship has the capacity to fully meet bids while also offering bids in return. This promotes depth and closeness while offering the nervous system and social brain the capacity to feel calm. It also feels safe and is not an immediate trigger when a bid is made and may be turned away on occasion. Usually, because there may be a repair to the missed bid down the road. Remember, it is not about perfection, but consistency. The attachment is secure, and no hard feelings are made. Additionally, this type of Reacher has the capacity to feel vulnerable because there is trust that the other person will also show vulnerability and reliability.

Some relationships can begin automatically secure, while others may take some time and effort to reach this space. Secure reaching can almost only be established with another secure Reacher. Reciprocated engagement creates depth, relational satisfaction, and bonding in relationships. This can also create positive beliefs of "I feel seen, heard, or acknowledged," or "I am valued and appreciated," resulting in healing components and protective factors against negative self-perceptions.

People may be Secure Reachers in some relationships and collapsed, vigilant, or mobilized in others. Secure reaching can emerge later in life through relationships that consistently offer safety and repair, even if early experiences were marked by inconsistency or unsafety. This doesn't mean reaching more; it means the other person needs to reciprocate and be intentional in how they meet your bids consistently.

Core experience: This pattern protects connection by trusting reciprocity:

- *Reaches with openness rather than caution.*
- *Expects emotional availability without demanding it.*
- *Feels comfortable expressing needs and receiving responses.*
- *Does not feel responsible for carrying connection alone.*
- *Experiences closeness as settling rather than effortful.*
- *Enforces positive beliefs.*

Supporting Research: Secure Reaching

Research across attachment theory, developmental psychology, and neuroscience consistently shows that secure attachment develops when bids for connection are met with sufficient responsiveness, predictability, and emotional attunement over time. In attachment research, securely attached individuals tend to use flexible strategies rather than rigid protective ones. They are able to seek support when needed, tolerate temporary misattunement, and return to connection without excessive vigilance or withdrawal (Mikulincer & Shaver, 2016; Fraley & Shaver, 2000).

Crucially, secure attachment does not require constant responsiveness. Instead, it emerges when caregivers or partners are reliably available, repair misattunements, and respond in ways that help the nervous system settle rather than escalate or shut down. From an emotion regulation perspective, people with histories of consistent emotional responsiveness are less likely to rely on suppression or hyperactivation. They show greater emotional flexibility, meaning they can express, modulate, and recover from emotional experiences without losing access to connection (Gross, 2015).

From a nervous system lens, reciprocal reaching reflects frequent access to the social engagement system. When the body has learned that reaching is met with safety, tone, eye contact, and presence often enough, it does not need to stay mobilized or conserve energy. Connection becomes regulating rather than dysregulating (Porges, 2011). Secure reaching is not permanent and not global. In other words, secure reaching is relationally earned, not biologically guaranteed.

Reflections

You might take a moment to notice your own patterns:

- *When bids don't land, do you reach less, reach more, or stay alert and waiting?*

- *Do you notice yourself conserving energy, escalating effort, or scanning for availability?*

- *Which pattern feels most familiar right now?*

- *Have these patterns shown up differently across relationships?*

- *What might this way of reaching be protecting you from?*

These patterns didn't develop randomly. They formed in response to what people and connection offered you in return over time.

Hard Truth

Some relationships may never offer the consistency or emotional availability required for reciprocal engagement. In those cases, it is important to understand what steps and conversations are necessary to promote healthy alignment from both parties. Sadly, and this is the hardest part we must face, the question becomes, "How do I protect myself from Contact Loneliness if the person just will not reciprocate?" At some point, we are responsible for our emotional responses, and after reading this, you now have increased awareness and responsibility for your role in this suffering.

I wish I could tell you that the person you want to hold on to the most will reciprocate, and I truly hope this book offers both of you just enough awareness to try. However, there will likely be individuals who will not reciprocate, and you must make a choice. "Do I continue holding on to a relationship where my bids will continue to go unmet, causing me to feel lonely in this relationship, or do I let go?" "Do I knowingly hold on to this pain and grieve the loss of what I hoped to get from this relationship, or face the grief of not having this person in my life?" Either way, grief is inevitable.

At the same time, when connection is met with enough presence, timing, and safety, reaching can shift. People can move toward Secure Reaching, a way of reaching that feels more open, flexible, and trusting, without needing to withdraw, escalate, or stay vigilant. Secure reaching isn't something you force or earn through effort. It emerges naturally over time when connection becomes reliably responsive enough for the body to relax.

Throughout this book, you may have noticed how often I reference the body or the nervous system. Before we discuss the necessary ingredients to a fully met bid, let's understand a little more deeply how the nervous system factors into bids. This will help explain why some people are more or less able to fully meet bids depending on their nervous system state.

Chapter 5

Three Nervous System States (Polyvagal)

I want to pause here and show you my appreciation for making it this far. Please bear with me, as this chapter might be a bit dense, but it is necessary to really understand why someone may biologically be unable to meet certain bids. Most people understand the nervous system as fight or flight, which alters how we interact in certain moments. What most people don't know is all the internal moving parts that become activated during this state.

Let's say you are walking down the street and, out of nowhere, a dog starts to chase you. Your nervous system will then shift into fight or flight to give you the resources, such as adrenaline, increased heart rate, and energy, to run or fight as a means of survival. However, there are other ways in which the nervous system becomes activated that are not life or death situations. These can occur during basic interactions at work, with a partner, with family, or in conversations with friends. There is a finite amount of emotional, mental, and physical energy or availability that we carry throughout the day. Once it is exhausted, our nervous system is essentially tapped out, making it harder to regulate, stay calm, or remain patient. This is important because once the nervous system is exhausted or in survival mode, it requires regulation or co regulation, an interactive process with a calm individual, rather than connection. Let's discuss the three phases of the nervous system and how they impact our overall behavioral capacity.

Polyvagal theory describes how the nervous system continuously shifts between states of safety and protection based on perceived cues in the environment and in relationships (Porges, 2011). This happens naturally, and we can shift between protection and safety throughout our day. These shifts are automatic and occur below conscious awareness. There are three stages: Ventral, Sympathetic, and Dorsal. Think about this like a traffic light. Green indicates a ventral state, meaning we are good to go and able to connect. Yellow means warning, as we are in a sympathetic fight or flight mobilized response. I like to think of it as, oh, it's yellow, let me floor it. Finally, we have red, the dorsal state, which is full shutdown and immobilization, meaning we are completely stopped.

Ventral Vagal (Safety and Connection)

This is the state of regulation and social engagement. When the ventral vagal system is active, the body feels safe enough to connect. Another important term to discuss here is the *window of tolerance*, which refers to how much ventral energy or capacity a person has. In this state, people can be emotionally present, flexible, curious, and responsive. Eye contact, tone of voice, facial expression, and shared attention come online naturally. This is the state where reciprocal engagement, bonding, and repair are most possible. Connection feels settling rather than effortful. Making bids and receiving bids feels easier and is more positively received.

Sympathetic (Mobilization and Protection)

This state activates when the nervous system detects threat, urgency, or uncertainty and is no longer in connection, but protection mode. The body mobilizes for action and moves into fight or flight. Emotionally, this can show up as anxiety, agitation, frustration, overexplaining, urgency to fix, or heightened effort to connect. While people may still seek connection in this state, it often feels driven, tense, or exhausting rather than calm and mutual. Connection feels urgent or effortful.

Dorsal Vagal (Shutdown and Conservation)

This state emerges when the nervous system perceives threat as overwhelming or inescapable. Energy drops. This state can also become activated during recurring unresolved conflict that feels hopeless or helpless. The body conserves by shutting down. Emotionally, this can look like withdrawal, numbness, collapse, hopelessness, or emotional disconnection. Reaching for connection may feel impossible or unsafe because the body is protecting itself and has turned the social engagement system offline. Making and receiving bids in this state can be detrimental, as it increases the risk of being met with a turn against response.

Social Engagement System & Window of Connection

Have you ever noticed your face go from smiling to flat depending on where you are or who you are with? Perhaps some days you are more open to engaging with others, and other days you just want to be in a dark room completely isolated. This is part of your *social engagement system*. There are moments when the body is more available for connection and moments when it is not. This is due to the social engagement system. The social engagement system refers to the part of the nervous system that allows us to feel safe enough to connect with others. When it is active, the body is more open to eye contact, tone of voice, facial expression, emotional presence, and reciprocal connection. In this state, we are better able to give and receive bids, respond flexibly, and feel emotionally accompanied.

The social engagement system comes online when the nervous system detects safety, and it goes offline when the body shifts into stress, threat, shutdown, or overload. Connection does not fail here because of a lack of care, but because the body no longer has the capacity to receive or offer it. The social engagement system lives in the ventral state described as the green light. Even a simple response offered during this state can settle us and help us feel less alone. The best interactions with another person happen when both social engagement systems are online. This creates what I call the *window of connection*, resulting in reciprocated engagement. The window of connection opens when both individuals are in a ventral state, and their social engagement systems are active. When the nervous system shifts into stress, shutdown, or overload, that receptivity narrows. The window of connection becomes smaller or may close altogether.

This shift can happen quickly and quietly. A person may look fine on the outside while their body has already moved into self-protection. A response offered when the social engagement system is open can land deeply. The same response, offered after the body has already braced, organized, or shut down, may be experienced as neutral or missed entirely. For example, if you are in a ventral state but the other person is in a dorsal state, you are in very different nervous system states, and bids are unlikely to be fully met. This is because the nervous system is no longer able to receive connection in the same way. In this sense, the window of connection reflects a brief overlap between emotional need and physiological readiness. When that overlap is missed, the moment passes, resulting in a missed connection or missed bid.

Alright, let's take a deep breath here, as we made it through that, and thank you for being patient. Now that we understand how the nervous system shapes availability for connection, we can finally dive into the three components that are essential to fully meeting bids. In the next chapters, we will explore how emotional presence and availability, emotional attunement, and timing shape whether connection lands or misses. Because connection does not fail for one reason alone.

Emotional Presence and Availability

When Someone Is There, but Not Fully with You

Have you ever felt like the person you are trying to connect with is physically present, but emotionally disengaged or absent? For example, maybe you are at a gathering and become playful, but your partner seems distant or disengaged. Physically, that person is present, but there is no emotional availability. Presence is more than just showing up or saying yes. It is the felt sense that someone is intentionally, emotionally, and attentively with you in the moment. Availability is about capacity. We often assume that if someone loves us, values us, or intends to be supportive, they should be able to meet us emotionally when we reach. When they cannot, it is easy to interpret that as disinterest, rejection, or lack of care. Not all but many moments of missed connection are about the limits of a person's nervous system.

This section recognizes how some individuals may be emotionally absent, and one key factor is their nervous system's capacity, often referred to as the window of tolerance. Many people have different ranges of mental, physical, or emotional bandwidth. Think of it this way: some green lights last longer than others, while some shift quickly to yellow. The window of tolerance refers to the range of nervous system activation in which a person can stay emotionally present, regulated, and responsive while remaining in a ventral state. When someone is within their window of tolerance, they can think clearly, feel emotions without becoming overwhelmed or shut down, and engage in connection with flexibility. When a person moves outside this window into states of hyperarousal, such as sympathetic activation marked by anxiety, agitation, or urgency, or hypoarousal, such as dorsal activation marked by numbing, withdrawal, or collapse, their capacity for connection, presence, and reciprocal engagement becomes limited. Some individuals may become overstimulated very quickly, while others may have a higher threshold for various stressors. Another example includes introverts versus extroverts, as they have different social tolerances and window of tolerance based on environment.

Additional factors such as stress, fatigue, distraction, overwhelm, emotional shutdown, and preoccupation also shape how available a person can be. Someone may deeply want to meet you and still not have the internal space to do so. For example, if one person's emotional bandwidth is at ten percent and the Reacher is at eighty percent, it is likely that they are not within the window of connection because one person is outside their window of tolerance. Therefore, if the Reacher makes a playful bid outside this window, it is likely to be met with an underwhelming response or risk a turn away or turning against response, resulting in a missed bid.

One day, I was with a friend, and we decided to go to a music festival. It started out great, and we were having fun. As time passed, I noticed that I was becoming more energized, while my friend was slowly depleting and becoming overstimulated. Within a few hours, our window of connection had closed, as I remained in a ventral state and my friend had shifted into a sympathetic state. I was enjoying the moment and trying to encourage my friend to dance and get excited with me, but my efforts were met with flat responses and frustration. Eventually, the window of connection fully closed. This resulted in me feeling lonely because we were no longer sharing the same presence. My friend was still physically there, but once they reached a dorsal state, they were emotionally shut down.

Their nervous system may have been overloaded. Their body may have been in a state of survival rather than openness. From the outside, this can look like flat responses, reduced expressiveness, or subtle distance, because the social engagement system is offline, causing facial muscles and tone of voice to become flatter.

Overall, when one person is in hyperarousal or hypoarousal, that individual is physiologically incapable of connecting and matching bids. Instead, the individual must focus on regulating or co regulating rather than connecting. It is imperative that the person outside the window of tolerance regulates before making further efforts to connect to prevent missed bids that can lead to contact loneliness. Unfortunately, in some relationships, certain lifestyles may contribute to how often the relationship remains in survival or protection mode. As a result, bids are more likely to be missed, leading to deeper relational complications. If a relationship stays in this state for prolonged periods of time, it can have significantly negative impacts, including emotional disconnection, resentment, frustration, and feeling lonely within the relationship.

Reflections

You might take a moment to notice how presence and availability show up in your relationships:

- *Are there people who respond reliably, but still feel emotionally distant?*

- *Can you think of moments when someone's presence, even briefly, made a meaningful difference?*

- *When others reach for you, how available do you tend to feel in your body?*

- *Are there times when you want to be present, but simply do not have the capacity?*

Sometimes a missed bid is not about emotional capacity, but attunement. They may simply not match the tone or intensity of the bid. Let's explore that next.

Emotional Energy & Attunement

When Emotional Expression Fails to Match

Have you ever shared something that mattered to you and felt disappointed almost immediately, not because the other person said anything wrong, but because the response did not quite fit the moment or match what you were offering? Maybe you walked away thinking, they responded, so why do I still feel off? Often, what is missing in these moments is a reciprocated response that aligns with the equivalent emotional energy.

Every bid carries an emotional tone and intensity. When we reach for connection, we are not only offering words; we are offering a feeling. And we are hoping, often unconsciously, that the other person will meet us at a similar emotional level. Matching energy does not mean matching words. It means matching the emotional temperature of the moment. For this section, it is more about how the receiver shows up physically and expressively, through body language, to match the emotional energy.

For example, imagine sharing something exciting and being met with a distracted nod. Or opening up about something painful and being met with quick reassurance or problem solving. On the surface, these responses may seem responsive or appropriate. However, they are missing emotional alignment. The response does not quite meet the feeling that was offered.

One Sunday after church, my mom and I were waiting in the lobby area for my little brother to come out of his class with all the other kids. As I watched the kids come out, I also noticed the parents talking to one another. The kids were so excited, running out with the drawings they had made during class. I could not help but notice one child who was eager to show his mom his drawing, but she was so distracted by another conversation that she turned to him, nodded, said that is nice, and immediately turned back to the other parent. The child looked a bit sad, so I asked my mom that when my little brother came out, she really gets excited with him about his drawing. I was a young teen at the time, and I did not really understand what I was asking my mom to do. Now, I understand how matching emotional energy with our bodies and facial expressions completes the bid by allowing the other person to feel seen.

When energy is matched, the experience feels different. The response feels aligned, resulting in emotional connection and a sense of being joined rather than redirected or dismissed. Even when the words are simple, the emotional presence feels right for the moment. This includes body language. It is not always about what is said, but how it is said. Body language plays an important role in emotional attunement because it offers a sense of feeling felt. It can include mirroring or facially matching the other person.

If the Reacher is excited and your face also lights up, subconsciously the Reacher will feel aligned in the bid. Similarly, if the bid comes from a place of fear, sadness, or anxiety, the receiver can adjust body language and tone of voice to help the Reacher feel seen and heard. This is why one person can say very little and still leave you feeling deeply connected, while another can say all the right things and leave you feeling unseen. As previously mentioned, some people soften their bids, lowering emotional intensity to avoid disappointment, often seen in Collapsed reaching. Others over explain, hoping clarity will help the response land, which is often seen in Mobilized reaching. Some stay alert and waiting, hoping the next moment will be different, which is common in Vigilant reaching.

Reflections

You might take a moment to notice how energy and safety show up in your own interactions:

- *When you share something meaningful, what kind of response helps your body feel settled?*

- *Are there times when you lower your emotional intensity to match others?*

- *Do you notice moments when someone matches your energy so naturally that you feel relief afterward?*

- *How do you tend to respond when someone brings strong emotion to you? Do you lean in, redirect, or pull back?*

In the next chapter, we will explore another factor in connection: timing. Because even a well-intended, emotionally aligned response can miss if it arrives outside the moment the nervous system was ready to receive it

Chapter 8

Timing Matters

When Connection Arrives Too Early or Too Late

Finally, we have timing. Have you ever reached out to someone or made the effort, but the response came too late? There are moments when someone responds with care, attention, and good intention, yet the response still does not land. The words and tone may be kind, and still the feeling remains because it was past the moment when it was needed most. Timing matters more than we often realize.

When we reach for connection, we are offering a moment in time. When connection arrives after the window of connection has closed, it can still be appreciated, but it often cannot do the same work. The nervous system has already shifted. The reach has already been tucked away. This does not mean late responses are uncaring. It means the body experiences connection in real time, and if delayed, it results in a missed bid. It is important to note that when Secure Reachers are consistently reciprocated, even if a response is delayed, it is still deemed safe to receive a delayed response on occasion.

However, repeated experiences like this begin to shape how people reach for connection. Some stop sharing unless something feels urgent. Some wait until they can organize their feelings perfectly before speaking. Some stop expecting emotional presence in the moment altogether. Timing may not always align. Life happens, or people are working or tired. When connection arrives within the window often enough, trust builds due to reliability. The body learns that reaching is worth it. When it rarely does, people adapt by reaching less, reaching differently, or expecting less.

One afternoon, when I was a young teen, I asked my dad if he would play basketball with me, and he said he was busy and it was not a good time. I got sad, but it made sense. A few hours passed, and I noticed he was playing with my sister. I got sadder. It was not that he did not want to play with me, but at the time I made my bid, he really was busy. My sister happened to ask him at a better timeframe, and it worked out for her. My dad's intention was not to make me feel bad, but he also failed to circle back to make a repair for the missed bid. The point is that sometimes we make bids that just will not be a good time for the other person, and there is no one to blame for this. Life happens, and we become preoccupied, or there are other things that are more urgent. If you try to make a bid as someone is heading out the door, chances are it is not a good time.

It is important to recognize that timing is not only about responses that come too late. Sometimes responses come too quickly, before the feeling has fully formed, before the person has finished reaching. Advice offered too soon, redirecting the conversation to something else about them, reassurance given too fast, or humor used to move past discomfort can all feel dismissive to the emotional tone. In those moments, the person who reached may feel rushed, redirected, or subtly unseen because the moment needed more time and space for full expression. Note, if timing was a factor in a missed bid, it is the receiver's responsibility to circle back to the Reacher and make a repair; this will promote secure reaching.

Reflections

You might take a moment to notice how timing shows up in your own interactions:

- *When you share something meaningful, what kind of timing helps you feel settled?*

- *Do you notice moments when a response comes too late or too quickly?*

- *Are there people with whom your window of connection or timing feels naturally met?*

- *How does your body feel when a response lands at the right time, relief, ease, warmth?*

- *How does your body respond when it does not?*

These reflections are simply about noticing how timing, readiness, and connection move through your relationships. In the next chapter, we will bring all these pieces together and look at what happens when connection repeatedly misses despite care and intention. This is where the Engagement Erosion Loop begins to form, showing how small, moment to moment misses quietly accumulate into distance, adaptation, and relational loneliness.

The Engagement Erosion Loop

Now that you understand what a bid is, how the nervous system filters connection, the reaching types, and the BRR model of the three ingredients to bid reciprocity, we can discuss the loop that leads to Contact Loneliness. Have you ever looked at your relationship and thought, we are still together, we still talk, we still share life, so why do I feel so far away? This question often arises in the quiet spaces between interactions. Nothing has necessarily ended, and yet something essential feels thinner than it once did.

The Engagement Erosion Loop describes the gradual process by which emotional connection weakens over time when bids for connection are consistently responded to but not emotionally met. As described in the BRR model, emotional connection erodes from repeated misses in reciprocity and not from lack of contact. Rather than breaking through conflict or neglect, the loop forms through repeated near misses in energy, timing, or presence. Additionally, the more factors missing in a bid, the bigger the negative impact. As these moments accumulate, the nervous system adapts by conserving, escalating, or staying vigilant, subtly reshaping how a person reaches for connection. The relationship may remain active and intact, yet the felt sense of closeness diminishes, leading to Contact Loneliness within ongoing interaction.

The loop begins subtly and slowly. A bid is made, and the other person responds, but the response misses what the moment needed. When this happens repeatedly, the nervous system starts to learn that reaching may not bring relief. Similarly to the BBR model, the Engagement Erosion Loop also has its set of components. Here are the eight phases of the Engagement Erosion Loop.

Step One: A Bid Is Made

Someone reaches for connection, such as a comment, look, touch, or meme. At this stage, the body is open, and the nervous system is testing whether connection is available.

Step Two: The Bid Is Responded To, but Not Fully Met

The other person responds by turning towards, but something is missing. Timing is off, emotional energy does not match, or presence feels partial. There is no rejection, and interaction continues, but the body notices the difference between being answered and being met.

Step Three: The Nervous System Registers the Miss

Even when the mind explains it away, the nervous system records the experience. It notes whether the interaction felt settling or effortful, whether connection relieved something or added strain. This happens below conscious awareness. The body begins to associate reaching with uncertainty rather than ease.

Step Four: Subtle Adaptation Begins

After repeated near misses, the body starts to adjust. Reaching becomes more cautious, and bids become smaller, delayed, or more strategic. Emotional effort is recalculated to reduce emotional cost.

Step Five: Reaching Patterns Solidify

Over time, adaptation takes shape. Some people reach less to conserve, collapsed. Some reach harder to try to secure connection, mobilized. Some stay alert and waiting, unable to relax into closeness, vigilant. These patterns are protective responses, not personality traits. They reflect how connection has been experienced; not how much it is desired.

Step Six: Connection Becomes Functional Rather Than Nourishing

The relationship begins to function in autopilot. People talk and life is shared, but emotional depth thins and vulnerability is postponed. Conversations and presence become intermittent. The relationship still exists, but the feeling of being emotionally held becomes less familiar.

Step Seven: Contact Loneliness Settles In

Loneliness emerges from the accumulation of near missed bids, from being almost met again and again. The person may feel confused by their own experience because nothing appears wrong. And yet, the body feels alone inside connection. Negative emotions such as frustration, anger, disappointment, resentment, and hopelessness begin to compile

Step Eight: The Loop Reinforces Itself

Because reaching now feels riskier or more effortful, bids decrease or change. Fewer opportunities for being met occur. This reinforces the nervous system's belief that connection is unreliable. The loop continues unless something interrupts it. Overall, lashing out or stonewalling becomes prominent eroding the connection and resulting in disconnected relationships.

People may begin to:

- *Stop bringing up emotional topics.*

- *Share only after careful internal calculation.*

- *Reach less spontaneously.*

- *Carry emotional experiences privately.*

- *Feel lonelier despite continued interaction.*

Once the Engagement Erosion Loop has taken hold, relationships often change, and frustration and emotional pain increase. Connection becomes more functional than nourishing. Conversations may continue, but emotional depth decreases. Bids become smaller, more practical, or less frequent, and vulnerability is delayed or avoided. The relationship becomes thin, and it shifts toward having distance rather than depth leaving the relationship vulnerable and exposed. This can lead to the Reacher to find ways to cope with the loneliness and lack of reciprocity by searching for connection outside of the relationship.

Sadly, and the most confusing component, is that none of this requires major conflict, neglect, or lack of care. It develops through repeated near misses that teach the nervous system to conserve until Contact Loneliness takes over.

Reflections

You might take a moment to notice whether this loop feels familiar.

- *Do some connections feel more functional than emotionally nourishing?*

- *Do you immediately feel angry or frustrated and the intensity or the response may feel disproportionate ?*

- *Do you feel lonely with a specific person?*

In the next chapter, we will explore how this loop can begin to loosen through awareness, safety, and small shifts that allow connection to land again. When the nervous system begins to understand what has been happening, it can start making choices that protect against Contact Loneliness rather than silently adjusting to it. Because erosion happens slowly, and so does repair.

Chapter 10

Interrupting the Loop: Reaching for Healing

Well, here we are, finally. After a thorough understanding of how we got here, we now get to explore how to fix it. The truth is, if you are in this loop, I hope this gives you the tools to break it but know that it will take time and commitment from both parties. The Engagement Erosion Loop does not end with a dramatic moment because someone finally says the perfect thing or does everything right. More often, it begins to loosen when awareness and intention shift. The purpose of awareness is to help you recognize patterns without turning them into personal failures or villainizing someone. However, reminder that in some cases, if the receiver refuses accountability or willingness to explore ways to connect it can result in reinjury. Also, there is accountability in inaction, there may not be malicious intent, but lack of engagement from one person can still result in loneliness and disconnection. Remember it is important to establish safety first prior to making a bid for repair.

Think about it this way. Assume you injured your arm, but if you continue to use it, it will deter healing and potentially reinjure itself. The logical response is to give your arm the much-needed rest. Think about reaching the same way. The question then becomes, how do I heal loneliness internally or within myself? The answer is reciprocity while letting your bids for connection heal; be intentional who you bid to.

At the heart of restored bonding is reciprocity. Reciprocity means that emotional effort is met with emotional availability. Depending on the relationship, most relationships have a mutual responsibility to reciprocate to a certain extent. That reaching is met with presence and flows in both directions often enough to feel shared. When reciprocity is present, people do not have to overfunction or withdraw to protect themselves. They do not have to work so hard to maintain connection. The relationship itself begins to carry some of the weight. This does not mean relationships become easy. It means they become alive again. What this looks like is to stop reaching toward people who are not reciprocating engagement and being intentional with your bids until they feel safe enough to increase in frequency.

It is also important to recognize that interrupting the loop does not mean undoing the past. Your experience, effort, and adaptations are one hundred percent valid. It means noticing the present with a little more clarity and compassion. When people begin to understand why connection has felt difficult, why bids have not landed, why reaching has felt tiring, and why loneliness has grown quietly, the experience becomes less confusing, less self-blaming, and most importantly, less lonely.

Seeing the Pattern Without Blame

One of the most powerful interruptions to the Engagement Erosion Loop is recognizing that the distance did not come from a lack of care. It came from repeated moments where connection did not quite meet the nervous system's needs. When you see this, and begin externalizing the problem, the internal story often shifts from "What is wrong with me?" to "This makes sense." That shift alone can be regulating and grounding. It is important to note that this should not be utilized as justification, this does not apply to all relationships.

Instead of pushing yourself to reach more or shutting down completely, you may start to notice when reaching feels possible and when it does not. You may begin to trust your body's signals rather than override them. You may realize that some moments are better suited for connection than others and that this does not mean giving up. It means adjusting with intention. Here are the five steps to breaking the Engagement Erosion Loop in hopes of rekindling connection.

The Steps to Interrupting the Engagement Erosion Loop

Step One: Naming the Loop Without Blame

Awareness is the first interruption. Therefore, the first adjustment occurs when the pattern is named accurately and reframed. Be aware and label why the bid was a near miss and discuss with the other person how to adjust next time to increase connection. Explore together whether the bid was missed because of availability, emotional attunement, or timing.

Many people try to fix connection by focusing on behavior. But without understanding the loop, these efforts often reinforce it. When someone recognizes, "This is not about effort. This is about repeated emotional near misses," the nervous system often experiences immediate relief. Meaning making and accurate attribution reduce threat responses in the brain and decrease shame-based or self-blame, which otherwise keeps the nervous system mobilized or shut down, also known as "name it to tame it" (Siegel, 2012; Cozolino, 2014). Naming the loop creates safety before any behavior changes.

Step Two: Safety Before Connection

Regulation must come before repair. Connection cannot be repaired while one or both nervous systems are outside the window of tolerance. When people are activated, depleted, or shut down, bids are more likely to miss, even when intentions are good. Attempting emotional repair in these states often leads to further erosion. The relationship must feel emotionally, physically, and morally safe prior to making bids for connection. The receiver is also accountable to reciprocate. If unwilling, making bids should be postponed preventing further erosion.

Remember, the social engagement system is a prerequisite for reciprocal connection. Without ventral vagal activation, tone flattens, timing slips, and emotional attunement becomes biologically unavailable. Breaking the loop here begins by recognizing whether regulation is needed instead of connection. This may look like pausing a conversation, grounding the body, resting, or co regulating before returning to emotional content.

When connection feels safe, the ventral vagal system becomes more accessible. This supports eye contact, facial expressiveness, vocal tone, emotional attunement, and the ability to stay present with others. Social interaction begins to feel natural rather than effortful. This phase may take some time until safety is fully established. Please be mindful, if safety is not established, meaning one person is hostile, critical, unwilling to be open to accountability, bids should be postponed and additional interventions are necessary to prevent injury.

Step Three: Quantity of Reaching to Quality of Timing

Be very intentional with your reaching. This may initially feel counterintuitive, but less reaching offers the time to heal while increasing better moments. This is the healing component that prevents reinjury or retraumatizing experiences. Choose your bids with compassion. You might invest more energy where engagement feels reciprocal. You might need to set boundaries or abstain from making bids where connection repeatedly misses. Give yourself permission to rest instead of reaching when it feels unsafe. These choices do not need to be dramatic or justified. They simply reflect a growing respect for how connection works for you. Be mindful that as you reach less, some relationships may fade due to the lack of reciprocity. This can feel hurtful as well, so I encourage you to honor these feelings of grief as they come.

The most powerful change that interrupts erosion is not reaching more but reaching inside the window of connection. When bids are offered during moments of mutual availability, presence, and emotional capacity, even small responses can land deeply. This means having a conversation with each other to understand and learn about each other's window of tolerance. Be communicative and discuss when you're feeling tired, burned out, or anxious even if its unrelated to each other. It is important to do daily check-ins, so both parties are aware of the nervous system state and balance regulation and connection.

Research on attachment repair shows that timing and responsiveness, not frequency, predict felt security and trust (Mikulincer & Shaver, 2016; Simpson, 2017). Again, this step may feel counterintuitive, especially for Mobilized or Vigilant Reachers, because it may feel like letting go of connection. But reducing effort while increasing timing allows the nervous system to experience success again. The body begins to relearn, "When I reach, it is received."

Step Four: Creating New Experiences of Being Met

Repair requires repetition, not perfection. The nervous system does not change through a single moment of being met. It changes through consistent enough experiences that contradict and overwrite the old pattern. Even brief moments of emotional attunement, when repeated, rebuild trust in connection. Neuroscience research shows that repeated experiences of attuned interaction strengthen social neural networks and increase oxytocin release, reinforcing bonding and approach motivation (Cozolino, 2014; Siegel, 2012). Moments of emotional attunement activate bonding neurochemistry, including oxytocin and endogenous opioids. Oxytocin is also known as the "love hormone" which promotes emotional closeness and buffers the sympathetic nervous system. These chemicals reinforce feelings of warmth, trust, and closeness. Importantly, they also teach the brain that connection is rewarding and regulating.

This means that the bonding hormones and neurochemical responses within the body are stimulated again, rekindling motivation and excitement for connection. Repair does not require dramatic conversations or emotional breakthroughs. It requires frequent moments where energy is matched, timing is respected, and presence is felt. Over time, these moments weaken the erosion loop and strengthen secure reaching.

Step Five: Secure Reaching Emerges

Security is an outcome, not a demand. As the loop is interrupted, reaching begins to feel different. The nervous system becomes less preoccupied with monitoring for rejection or misattunement. The body no longer needs to brace. Emotional openness becomes safer because the expectation of being met outweighs the fear of being missed. Secure reaching emerges naturally when the nervous system no longer needs protection. Attachment research consistently shows that secure strategies are flexible, context sensitive, and experience dependent (Fraley & Shaver, 2000; Mikulincer & Shaver, 2016). This means security can grow later in life within specific relationships when emotional reciprocity becomes reliable enough.

Therefore, secure reaching is not forced but earned through reciprocated experiences. When connection has been reliably responsive, people can tolerate misattunement without collapsing, escalating, or becoming vigilant. Repair feels possible because the nervous system expects reconnection. Reaching feels open rather than cautious. Connection feels settling rather than effortful. The body trusts that bids will usually land or be repaired when they do not. This is how bonding is biologically maintained.

Reflections

You might take a moment to notice what interruption could look like for you:

- *What happens inside you when you recognize a pattern without judging it?*

- *Are there moments when reaching feels possible again, even briefly?*

- *How do you know when your body feels more open to connection?*

- *What would it be like to let those moments guide you, rather than forcing connection when it does not feel safe?*

Before closing this book, you might take one last moment to reflect.

- *What has felt most familiar as you have read these pages?*

- *What moments helped you feel seen?*

- *What understanding do you want to carry with you?*

You have been reaching for connection your whole life. Remember that reaching was never the problem. It was a sign of your capacity for care, attachment, and relationship. You do not need to reach differently today. You do not need to confront, explain, or decide. Connection does not return through effort alone. It returns when reaching begins to feel safe again. And that starts here, with noticing, with compassion, and with being met.

Chapter 11

For The Parents

This section may be hard for some parents. This is not about instilling guilt, shame, or stigma; it is about increasing awareness in order to restore connection with your children. Do you ever wonder if your child feels alone with you? A parent may be sitting nearby, responding when spoken to, or present in the room, yet the child's body senses something missing. Children don't experience connection through words alone. They experience it through patterns and play. Though children's bids may feel simple and for some unimportant, they notice how often someone responds, returns, and emotionally meets them when they reach out. These moments are usually small and ordinary. It may look like your child asking you to watch them do a flip, or to sit with them and draw. As a parent myself, I am well aware that sometimes these bids can be a bit let's say underwhelming. Nonetheless, for them, it means so much more. There is only so many, "watch this" that I can take, but I put on a smile and make sure she knows I'm present. This is the same form of affection we want from others; our children deserve the same in return.

From early development, children are wired to reach for connection. Long before language, they reach with eye contact, movement, sound, and proximity. Their nervous system notices if the parent showed up in an appropriate amount of time to provide food, warmth, or comfort. As they grow, these reaches become questions, stories, play invitations, emotional expressions, and bids for shared attention. When a caregiver notices and responds to these bids in a way that feels emotionally attuned, it promotes closeness and safety. The child's nervous system organizes around safety, and emotions feel more manageable. Over time, children begin to expect that connection involves mutual effort and shared presence.

Of course, parents have busy lives, and at times our responses may be delayed, distracted, or emotionally mismatched. The child doesn't usually interpret this cognitively or make sense of what just happened mentally. Unfortunately, children may not always express how a missed bid makes them feel, and can internalize the experience. Instead, they feel it somatically; their body registers the experience as uncertainty. Over time, repeated missed bids can teach a child that proximity does not guarantee connection, and that being physically together does not always mean being emotionally met.

Some children adapt by reaching louder, which may appear as acting out through physical aggression, emotional outbursts, or defiance. Others adapt by reaching less, learning to manage their needs internally through withdrawal, minimization, or emotional suppression. When children begin to reach less, they may also reduce emotional expression, communicating in more passive or indirect ways. Still, others become highly attuned to those around them, carefully tracking moods, availability, and emotional shifts as a way to anticipate connection or disconnection. These patterns are not personality traits, but relational adaptations shaped by repeated experiences of how bids for connection are met or missed (Ainsworth et al., 1978; Cassidy & Shaver, 2016; Eisenberg et al., 2010; Tronick, 2007).

When bids are met consistently, children internalize a sense of relational safety. When bids are inconsistently met or met without emotional engagement children may begin to carry the emotional work of connection alone. Presence without engagement can feel confusing to a child's nervous system. The adult is there, yet something essential is missing. When this pattern becomes chronic, it may resemble what some have described as an emotionally absent parent.

It's important to recognize that no caregiver meets every bid. What matters is whether connection can be restored, repaired, and how often bids are fully met. Repair teaches something powerful: even when connection breaks, it can come back. Children don't need constant attention. They need responsive attention. Attention that communicates *I see you. I'm here. I'm trying.* Over time, these experiences shape how children approach relationships, express emotions, and interpret closeness. They influence whether reaching feels hopeful or risky, and whether connection feels mutual or one-sided.

Reflections

Before moving forward, you may want to pause and notice your own experiences of connection:

- *When you were a child, how were your bids usually met?*

- *Were there people who were physically present but emotionally unavailable?*

- *How did your body respond when you felt truly met versus when you didn't?*

You might also reflect on the children in your life.

- *How do they tend to reach for connection?*

- *Do their bids come through words, behavior, play, or emotion?*

- *Have you asked them how they feel when you miss a bid?*

Finally, you may notice your own responses:

- *When a child reaches for you, how available do you tend to be in that moment?*

- *Are there times when you want to meet them more fully but feel limited by stress, fatigue, or distraction?*

- *How does it feel in your body when you're able to truly meet a child, and when you're not?*

At the end of this book, I have included an adapted Reciprocity of Engagement Scale to help assess the relational experience between you and your child. It can be difficult for some parents if their child scores the relationship low. My hope is that this information is received with compassion and openness, allowing space for meaningful change, repair, and deeper connection so your child can truly feel seen by you.

Final Thoughts

I want to make something extremely clear. You are not dramatic. You are not needy. You are not asking for too much. Wanting emotional connection is a human biological necessity. It is attachment. It is your nervous system doing exactly what it was designed to do, reaching toward safety, closeness, and belonging.

Contact Loneliness can be one of the hardest experiences to explain because, on the outside, the relationship may look fine. People are still there, hanging out and doing things. Communication might even be consistent. And yet, something inside you continues to feel a sense of emptiness. What you have been feeling is real and not a personality flaw. It is a nervous system response to repeated moments of being almost met.

If this book gave you anything, I hope it gave you language and a new way of understanding and expressing your frustrations, needs, and wants. Language for the difference between being responded to and being emotionally met. Language for the way timing, energy, and presence shape whether connection lands. Language for the adaptations you developed to protect yourself from the emotional cost of reaching.

You deserve a reciprocated relationship that promotes emotional depth. I hope it also gave you permission to stop blaming yourself for needing more than surface-level interaction. Permission to respect your body's signals when connection feels unsafe or inconsistent. Permission to grieve what you hoped a relationship would become, even if it never turned into that. And permission to move toward relationships where reciprocity is felt, not just promised.

You should not feel as if you must force connection or chase emotional availability. You do not have to work twice as hard to be met halfway. Healing begins when your nervous system no longer feels like it must earn closeness through effort, silence, or endurance. You have been reaching for connection your whole life. That reaching was never the problem. It was always proof of your desire to love and feel loved.

Unfortunately, loving someone is not enough. It requires consistent, reciprocated effort to show up mutually for each other. The goal is not to become someone who needs less or to lose yourself by giving up parts of who you are. The goal is to build a life where what you need is met with enough presence, enough consistency, and enough care. A life in which relationships no longer feel lonely but bonded through reciprocated nurturing.

Reflection & Journal Section

1. Noticing How You Reach

Take a moment to reflect on how you tend to reach for connection.

- *When I want to feel closer to someone, what do I usually do?*

- *Do my bids tend to be direct, subtle, playful, practical, emotional, or quiet?*

- *Have I learned to soften, shrink, explain, or wait before reaching?*

- *Are there relationships where reaching feels easier and others where it feels heavier?*

2. Being Responded To vs. Being Met

Think about recent interactions.

- *Can I recall a time when someone responded, but I still felt unseen?*

- *What was missing in that moment energy, timing, presence, or something else?*

- *Can I remember a time when I felt emotionally met, even briefly?*

- *What did my body feel like afterward?*

3. Your Reaching Pattern(s)

Many people recognize themselves in more than one pattern.

- *When bids don't land, do I tend to:*
  - *reach less (collapsed),*
  - *reach harder (mobilized),*
  - *or stay alert and waiting (vigilant)?*
- *Do different relationships bring out different patterns in me?*
- *What do these patterns seem to be protecting me from?*

4. Safety and Capacity

Pause here if this feels tender.

- *Are there relationships where reaching hasn't felt safe?*
- *Have there been moments when my needs were used against me, dismissed, or ignored?*
- *How has my body learned to protect itself in those environments?*
- *What does "emotional safety" feel like for me when it's present?*

5. Energy, Timing, and Presence

Reflect on moments of connection that *did* land.

- *When someone meets my energy, how does my body respond?*
- *When timing feels right, what changes inside me?*
- *How do I know when someone is truly present with me?*
- *How available do I tend to feel when others reach for me?*

6. The Engagement Erosion Loop

Gently consider whether you recognize this pattern.

- *Have I noticed myself adapting how I reach over time?*

- *Are there relationships that feel more functional than nourishing?*

- *Do I ever stop myself from sharing without fully knowing why?*

- *What happens in my body when I imagine reaching again?*

7. Moments of Being Met

This section is about remembering not longing.

- *When have I felt emotionally met in my life?*

- *What made those moments feel different?*

- *How did my body respond before, during, and after?*

- *What did those moments teach me about what connection can feel like?*

8. Carrying This Forward

As you close this section, you might ask yourself:

- *What feels clearer now than it did before?*

- *What do I trust about my experience that I didn't trust before?*

- *Where might I want to be gentler with myself?*

- *What does "enough connection" look like for me right now?*

The Reciprocity of Engagement Scale

Throughout this book, we've talked about reaching, bids, and what it feels like to be emotionally met or almost met. We've explored how Contact Loneliness doesn't come from a lack of people, but from a lack of reciprocal emotional engagement. Many readers ask a natural question at this point:

"How do I know if what I'm feeling is real?" "How do I tell the difference between a rough season and a relationship that consistently leaves me lonely?"

I created Reciprocity of Engagement Scale to help answer those questions. All scales can be downloaded for free from my website www.josegarciacuellar.com. This is not a diagnosing tool to assign blame, but to help you notice patterns over time throughout your relationships. This scale is not about proving that someone is "bad" or that a relationship has failed. It is about bringing clarity and confirmation to something that often stays vague and confusing. When connection feels off, people tend to turn inward and ask, "What's wrong with me?" This tool gently externalizes that question toward something more accurate: "What is actually happening between us?"

What the Scale Measures

The Reciprocity of Engagement Scale focuses on felt experience, not intention. It helps you notice:

- *Whether emotional effort flows in both directions.*

- *Whether bids are consistently met with presence, timing, and attunement.*

- *Whether you feel emotionally accompanied or emotionally alone after interactions.*

- *Whether connection feels settling or effortful over time.*

Importantly, this scale does not measure how much someone says they care, how long you've been together, or how often you communicate. Many relationships have frequent contact and still lack reciprocity of engagement. Additionally, this does not evaluate you but more so the other person within the relationship.

How to Use the Scale

Step 1: Choose One Relationship at a Time

Answer the scale with one specific relationship in mind (for example: a romantic partner, a close friendship, or a family relationship). Do not average multiple relationships together. Patterns are relational, not global or general.

Step 2: Answer Based on Experience, Not Hope

Respond based on what you experience most of the time, not what you wish were true and not the occasional high point. Try to stay within a month or specific scenario from that relationship.

If you notice yourself thinking: "Well, sometimes…" "They mean well…" "They're trying…" Pause, and return to: What does my body experience most often after I reach? Stay objective to the questions.

Step 3: Use Your Body as Information

As you answer each item, notice what happens inside you. Do you feel tension, relief, heaviness, or clarity? Your nervous system often recognizes patterns before your mind does. This scale works best when you let your first, honest response guide you.

What the Scores Mean

Rather than labeling relationships as healthy or unhealthy, the Reciprocity of Engagement Scale helps identify where engagement tends to break down.

- **Higher scores** suggest that emotional engagement is more consistently reciprocated. Reaching feels secure and safe. Connection tends to settle the nervous system rather than exhaust it.

- **Moderate scores** often reflect inconsistency. Bids are sometimes met and sometimes missed, which can lead to vigilance, confusion, or emotional fatigue.

- **Lower scores** suggest that emotional engagement is largely one-sided or unreliable. Reaching may feel effortful or risky, even if the relationship continues.

How to Hold What You Discover

After you add the scores divide by the number of questions, remember to reverse number 8 and 15 after you originally score it. Whatever your score, this scale is not asking you to confront, explain, or decide anything immediately. It is simply offering context and validation. Many people feel an unexpected sense of relief after completing the scale because the experience finally has language. Others may find it worrisome or concerning because it makes your experience real and though validating, it also confirms your fears. This can be a very difficult thing to face or accept. I truly hope this scale cannot just validate your experience but overall give you the language to open a conversation with that person and have a dialogue on what is really happening in that relationship.

Finally, if the scale highlights low reciprocity, it doesn't mean you should reach more. It means your body has likely been working very hard to stay connected. If it highlights higher reciprocity, it may help you recognize why certain relationships feel more nourishing, lighter, or safer to rest inside. Either way, awareness itself is already an interruption of the Engagement Erosion Loop. It should bring awareness to help you understand what has already been happening. You are allowed to want reciprocity. You are allowed to notice imbalance. And you are allowed to let information guide compassion for yourself first. Take this slowly. And trust what your body has been trying to tell you all this time.

Reciprocity of Engagement Scale (RES)

Instructions: "Think about your relationship over the past month or another specified period. "Partner" could mean (family member, friend, co-worker, romantic partner, etc.) Rate each statement from 0–4."

0 = Never, 1 = Rarely, 2 = Sometimes, 3 = Often, 4 = Almost always

Subscale A: Affective Attunement (AA)	
1. My partner's emotional tone matchesthe emotional tone of my bid.	
2. When I share something vulnerable,Ifeel emotionally *met*, not just acknowledged.	
3. My partner responds in a way thatfitsthe intensity of what I'm feeling.	

Subscale B: Contingency & Timing (CT)	
4. My partner respondswithin atime window that still feels connected to the moment.	
5. Even if my partner can't respond immediately, they return to the bid in a meaningful way.	
6. When my partner responds later than expected, the response still feels emotionally connected to my original bid.	

Subscale C: Attentional Presence (AP)	
7. My partner givesme real attention when I reach for connection.	
8. I feel like I'm competing with distractions (phone, tasks, etc.) when I bid. *(reverse)*	
9. My partner's response feels engaged rather than automatic.	

Subscale D: Co-regulatory Impact (CRI)	
10. After mypartnerresponds, I feel calmer or more grounded.	
11. My partner's responses help me feel safe and connected in my body.	
12. Even during stress, my partner's engagement helps us settle rather than escalate.	

Subscale E: Proportional Investment (PI)	
13. Mypartner's responsefeelsproportionate to the bid (not minimal or perfunctory).	
14. When I reach, my partner meets me with comparable effort.	
15. I feel like I carry the emotional "work" of connection alone. *(reverse)*	

Scoring
- Reverse-scoreitems **8** and **15** (0↔4, 1↔3, 2 stays 2).
- Compute:
  - **Total RES** =average of all items (0–4)
  - Subscaleaverages (AA, CT, AP, CRI, PI)

Interpretation
- **3.2–4.0** Highreciprocity: bids reliably become felt connection
- **2.4–3.1** Moderate/inconsistent: connection occurs but is fragile or uneven
- **1.6–2.3** Lowreciprocity: "acknowledged but not met" is common
- **0–1.5** Chroniclowreciprocity: strong risk for erosion loop/loneliness

© 2026 Dr. Jose Garcia-Cuellar. All rights reserved. www.josegarciacuellar.com
TheReciprocity of Engagement Scale(RES) wasdeveloped bythe authorof"WithYou, But Alone" for research and scholarly use. Permission is granted for use in research and clinical contexts with appropriate citation. Adaptation or commercial use requires written permission from the author.

Reciprocity of Engagement Scale- Parent/Caregiver *(RES-PC)*

(Parent/Caregiver) Instructions: "Think about your child's interactions with you (or the identified caregiver) over the past month. Rate how often each statement is true."

0 = Never, 1 = Rarely, 2 = Sometimes, 3 = Often, 4 = Almost always

Subscale A: Affective Attunement (AA)	
1. I match my child's emotional tone when they seek connection.	
2. When my child shares distress, they feel emotionally met rather than dismissed.	
3. My response fits the intensity of my child's emotional state.	

Subscale B: Responding & Coming Back (Contingency & Timing)	
4. I respond within a timeframe that still feels meaningful to my child.	
5. If I cannot respond immediately, I return to my child's bid later.	
6. When I return, my response remains emotionally connected to the original bid.	

Subscale C: Paying Attention (Attentional Presence)	
7. I give my child my full attention when they seek connection.	
8. My child competes with distractions (phone, tasks, etc.) for my attention. *(reverse)*	
9. My responses feel intentional and engaged rather than automatic.	

Subscale D: Feeling Calm & Safe (Co-regulatory Impact)	
10. My child appears calmer after connecting with me.	
11. My responses help my child feel physically and emotionally safe.	
12. During stress, our interaction tends to settle rather than escalate.	

Subscale E: Trying Together (Proportional Investment)	
13. My level of effort matches my child's bids for connection.	
14. When my child reaches for me, I meet them with comparable effort.	
15. My child carries most of the effort to stay emotionally connected. *(reverse)*	

Scoring
- Reverse-score items **8** and **15** (0↔4, 1↔3, 2 stays 2).
- Compute:
    - **Total RES** = average of all items (0–4)
    - Subscale averages (AA, CT, AP, CRI, PI)

Interpretation
- **3.2–4.0** High reciprocity: bids reliably become felt connection
- **2.4–3.1** Moderate/inconsistent: connection occurs but is fragile or uneven
- **1.6–2.3** Low reciprocity: "acknowledged but not met" is common
- **0–1.5** Chronic low reciprocity: strong risk for erosion loop/loneliness

© 2026 Dr. Jose Garcia-Cuellar. All rights reserved. www.josegarciacuellar.com
The Reciprocity of Engagement Scale (RES) was developed by the author of "With You, But Alone" for research and scholarly use. Permission is granted for use in research and clinical contexts with appropriate citation. Adaptation or commercial use requires written permission from the author.

Reciprocity of Engagement Scale- Young Child *(RES-YC)*

(Ages: 4-12) Instructions: "I'mgoing toreadsomesentences.Thinkabout when you try to talk, play, or get helpfromthisperson.Point totheface thatshowshowoftenthishappens."

Never   Almost never   Sometimes   A lot   Almost always
0=Never,1=Rarely,2=Sometimes,3=Often,4= Almostalways

Subscale A: Matching Feelings (Affective Attunement)	
1. When I feel happy or sad, this person notices my feelings.	
2. When I'm upset, this person tries to understand me.	
3. This person reacts in a way that fits how big my feelings are.	

Subscale B: Responding & Coming Back (Contingency & Timing)	
4. When I try to talk or play, thisperson responds soon.	
5. If they can't respond right away, they come back later.	
6. When they come back, they remember what I wanted or needed.	

Subscale C: Paying Attention (Attentional Presence)	
7. This person looks at me and listenswhen I try to connect.	
8. This person is busy with phones, screens, or other things when I want them. *(reverse)*	
9. This person's response feels real, not rushed.	

Subscale D: Feeling Calm & Safe (Co-regulatory Impact)	
10. After being with this person, my body feelscalmer.	
11. This person helps me feel safe when I'm upset.	
12. When things feel hard, being with this person helps me feel better.	

Subscale E: Trying Together (Proportional Investment)	
13. This persontries when I try to connect.	
14. We both work to stay connected.	
15. I feel like I'm the only one who tries to connect. *(reverse)*	

Scoring

- Reverse-scoreitems **8** and **15** (0↔4, 1↔3, 2 stays 2).
- Compute:
  - **Total RES** =average of all items (0–4)
  - Subscaleaverages (AA, CT, AP, CRI, PI)

Interpretation

- **3.2–4.0** Highreciprocity: bids reliably become felt connection
- **2.4–3.1** Moderate/inconsistent: connection occurs but is fragile or uneven
- **1.6–2.3** Lowreciprocity: "acknowledged but not met" is common
- **0–1.5** Chroniclowreciprocity: strong risk for erosion loop/loneliness

© 2026 Dr. Jose Garcia-Cuellar. All rights reserved. www.josegarciacuellar.com
TheReciprocity of Engagement Scale(RES) wasdeveloped bythe authorof"WithYou, But Alone" for research and scholarly use. Permission is granted for use in research and clinical contexts with appropriate citation. Adaptation or commercial use requires written permission from the author.

Reference

Ainsworth, M. D. S., Blehar, M. C., Waters, E., & Wall, S. (1978). *Patterns of attachment: A psychological study of the strange situation*. Hillsdale, NJ: Erlbaum.

Cassidy, J., & Shaver, P. R. (2016). *Handbook of attachment: Theory, research, and clinical applications* (3rd ed.). New York, NY: Guilford Press.

Eisenberg, N., Spinrad, T. L., & Eggum, N. D. (2010). Emotion-related self-regulation and its relation to children's maladjustment. *Annual Review of Clinical Psychology, 6*, 495–525. https://doi.org/10.1146/annurev.clinpsy.121208.131208

Fraley, R. C., & Shaver, P. R. (2000). Adult romantic attachment: Theoretical developments, emerging controversies, and unanswered questions. *Review of General Psychology, 4*(2), 132–154. https://doi.org/10.1037/1089-2680.4.2.132

Gottman, J. M., Coan, J., Carrere, S., & Swanson, C. (1998). Predicting marital happiness and stability from newlywed interactions. *Journal of Marriage and the Family, 60*(1), 5–22. https://doi.org/10.2307/353438

Gross, J. J. (2015). Emotion regulation: Current status and future prospects. *Psychological Inquiry, 26*(1), 1–26. https://doi.org/10.1080/1047840X.2014.940781

Günaydin, G., Selçuk, E., & Ong, A. D. (2021). Perceived partner responsiveness fluctuations promote attachment anxiety. *Journal of Personality and Social Psychology, 121*(4), 695–718. https://doi.org/10.1037/pspi0000337

Horowitz, L. M. (2004). *Interpersonal foundations of psychopathology*. American Psychological Association. https://doi.org/10.1037/10727-000

Mikulincer, M., & Shaver, P. R. (2016). *Attachment in adulthood: Structure, dynamics, and change* (2nd ed.). Guilford Press.

Porges, S. W. (2011). *The polyvagal theory: Neurophysiological foundations of emotions, attachment, communication, and self-regulation*. W. W. Norton & Company.

Siegel, D. J. (2012). *The developing mind: How relationships and the brain interact to shape who we are* (2nd ed.). Guilford Press.

Simpson, J. A. (2017). Adult attachment, stress, and romantic relationships. *Current Opinion in Psychology, 13*, 19–24. https://doi.org/10.1016/j.copsyc.2016.04.006

Tronick, E. (2007). *The neurobehavioral and social-emotional development of infants and children*. New York, NY: W. W. Norton & Company.

Whitchurch, E. R., Wilson, T. D., & Gilbert, D. T. (2011). "He loves me, he loves me not…": Uncertainty can increase romantic attraction. *Psychological Science, 22*(2), 172–175. https://doi.org/10.1177/0956797610393745

www.ingramcontent.com/pod-product-compliance
Lightning Source LLC
Chambersburg PA
CBHW031500150726
47990CB00007B/2830